Chapter 1 Baby B

On a bitter January night, I awaken to the sound of screaming. As my heart races and I struggle to focus, there is an urgent need to fly out of bed toward the emergency. Something horrific is happening. As I begin to gain my senses, I realize it is my son James yelling that his brother Ryan is having a seizure. The twins are 12 years old and share a bedroom.

I race to their bedroom to look towards the bottom bunk where I see Ryan convulsing in his bed. The only light in the room is the light coming from his hand-held device. I feel the color drain from my face as I attempt to wrap my head around what is happening. My 16-year-old daughter is on the phone calling for an ambulance as I attend to my son. I feel helpless as I have no idea what to do or how to handle the situation. The boy's father races into the room and calls Ryan's name to try to pull him out of the seizure to no avail.

The ambulance seems to take forever to arrive. In come the police and EMS crew to provide aide to my son. All I can do is move aside and watch. My pulse is racing while I am trying to understand and make sense of the situation. My head is reeling as I think about what the implications are for my son and whether he will be able to live a normal life. He is slow to come out of the seizure and the noises Ryan makes while attempting to recover brain function are quite unsettling. Unfortunately, it is something you can never forget.

The decision is made to transport him to the hospital. The emergency personnel wheel Ryan out of the house across the frozen front yard adorned with various Christmas decorations.

The hospital visit and testing do not really provide any answers other than a normal cat scan of the brain and a freak occurrence. Unbeknownst to me this is the start of a lifelong seizure journey. Ryan was previously diagnosed with ADHD as well as anxiety and depression and has been taking medications for those conditions for several years. Sleep has not come easy for him due to those medications and lack of sleep can be a contributing factor for seizures.

Ryan had always been a pleasant child however the school system was not his friend. Having ADHD has caused him to struggle with focus, often falling behind in his work and requiring frequent school meetings throughout the year. The educators would develop a treatment plan for the best way to help him learn. Children with ADHD can have behavior problems as they struggle to fit in and keep up with the tasks at hand. They often feel ostracized as they are given extra attention in school which creates a snowball effect.

Ryan was the epitome of oppositional defiance. His refusal to do certain things was off the charts. I always thought when he was young that he was very bright, more intelligent than most, however his condition did not support that. Now that he is older it is clear he is highly intelligent.

As Ryan's ADHD continued so did his anxiety and depression. By the time he was due to begin high school, he could not overcome his fears, and attendance would become a problem. He refused to go to school on his first day of high school, as he told me he had laid awake all-night thinking about hanging himself. This was devastating for me but more so for him. This precipitated a trip to an E.R where his shoelaces were removed, and a recommendation was given for inpatient treatment. Ryan was not at all on board with that and refused to stay. There was an alternative given which provided a day treatment program that would count as credit for school attendance as well as provide the needed therapy.

As a parent you will do anything to help your child succeed. I was working full time and taking care of 3 children as well as a home. I was able to adjust my hours so that I could provide the transportation Ryan needed to attend the outpatient program. He did not want to be caught dead on the "little white van" that the program provided. After several weeks this became too much for Ryan to handle and he began to refuse to go. No matter the threats or promises to take away his privileges he would not budge.

Eventually the school filed charges for truancy which just complicated everything and added additional stress. The charges were dismissed as the school representative had never laid eyes on Ryan and came unprepared. He looked like a fool. I made the decision to withdraw

him from the book and mortar public school in our township in favor of cyber school. A fresh start in a different environment with a lot of support from his new teachers, me myself and I, would save his education.

As a college graduate, I knew the importance of having a good education and how it could further you in life. I also knew it would be challenging for Ryan due to his condition and that he hated school and did not see the value of getting a good education.

Having children in cyber school while working can be a challenge as you call home to confirm the child is up and ready to log onto their school computers daily to frequently have your call go unanswered.

Chapter 2 Baby A

He came out screaming of course as he was only 4 pounds 1 ounce (about 29.57 ml). James wanted to make himself known and still does to this day! The twins were born at 36 weeks (about 8 and a half months) which was not too bad. However, I only gained 8 pounds; it was the only time in my life where I could not gain weight. Bed rest was mandatory at 7 or 8 months, and I developed gestational diabetes. This was difficult as I also had a 3-year-old daughter to care for.

With twin pregnancy ultrasounds are done more frequently. I was advised early on that James's stomach was underdeveloped or smaller than it should be. No wonder he vomited with such force for at least the first 5 years of his life. To this day he suffers from frequent heartburn, which I am sure is complicated by his diet.

The twins came home with heart monitors used for detection of infants who stop breathing or SIDS. I understand the importance of them but living through frequent alarms can be unnerving. After a couple of months, it was determined that no events had occurred so that the alarms were removed. Affixing the stickies on the chest of an exceedingly small baby is difficult as they had to be offset and their chest or abdomen areas are so small it is difficult to accomplish.

In the beginning, their dad and I switched off nights so that someone would sleep while the other did not at all. Babies that are small will eat an ounce every two hours. I remember saying it is only 14 feedings and 10 diaper changes per night, which was a nightmare. I preferred to feed them separately as opposed to simultaneously. When one was done the other would wake up. It was not until we split them up that thing became a little easier.

James was a sweet impish baby who was very affectionate and fun. He loved adventures and as he got older it continued. From riding big wheels to dirty bikes, he was in his glory. Always testing the limits and never wanting to follow the rules. James loved to push everyone and everything to see how far he could go.

As James began school, he faltered as he was often called out for behavior issues and needed more support for reading. Always they showoff but never in an effective way. He was diagnosed with ADD at one point but refused the medicine as he entered middle school. I never thought that paying attention was an issue for him. We were all looking for a diagnosis to help him become successful in school. His therapist at one point felt he may have a personality disorder.

James had frequent detentions on Saturdays, which punish the parents as it is one more day of fighting to get the child out of bed and to school on time. During his attendance at one of these detentions, he vandalized the school, resulting in charges and a hefty suspension. It was an expensive penalty with legal fees which we as parents incurred.

When high school began it was clear that the behavior issues continued. I would drop James off for school only to learn that he would go inside and then turn around and walk home as soon as I pulled away from the curb. It became clear that he did not value his education, so the decision was made to enroll him in cyber school. James is bright and creative as he excels in computer design and development.

James would stay up all night gaming and yelling only to realize the night had passed and he had to get some sleep before going to school. He developed networks of his own and would loan them to other online gaming associates for their use. This got him in a lot of trouble as one user took down several major company's websites using one of his servers, and yes it was traced back to him resulting in an FBI raid of our home. This is not an experience I would wish on anyone.

Chapter 3 The Parents

We met at a local diner. I had hung up my professional shoes and ended a 10-

year high school relationship. As I was out on my own, I needed fast money to handle my bills. I knew how to serve as I had done so during my teenage years. So, I headed to a local diner applied and was hired on the spot. The diner was run by an infamous Greek family that was quite colorful. From the hell-raising grandfather sitting in his chair at the front of the restaurant watching everyone and everything, to the entitled grandchildren with their fancy cars and better-than-thou attitude, it was an interesting place.

Most of the employees were high school educated or less, which created a diverse bunch. As a college graduate, I felt out of place. However, after ending a long-term relationship where I felt like I had missed my teens and early twenties, it was exactly what I needed. The bar scene became a regular part of my life encompassing many sleepless nights and matches not made in heaven. I was making up for lost time and having fun doing it. My coworkers and I quickly became friends and spent many hours clubbing and enjoying the "high life."

After a couple of years and in my mid-twenties I wanted to settle down, get married and have kids. The pickings in that lifestyle were slim and as a result I took the first person who latched onto me, who I felt had potential. The twin's dad was a regular customer at the diner as he worked across the street from the diner so I would see him daily. He was shy yet made his interest in me known. I was undecided as to whether I should go out with him, but he was persistent and eventually I did.

Our first date was to an annual residential weekend party. He picked me up in an old blue LTD and drove like a bat out of hell. I thought at the start of the date that I already wanted to go home. I had never been in a car with anyone who drove as if he were on a racetrack. No wonder as it turned out he had no license. The party was fun as they often are with unlimited drinks and drugs. What I have learned over the years is that these situations result in foggy evaluations of your life and your circumstances. Decisions cannot be made while in the party life mindset. Our first date ended with a bang and the rest is history. I ignored my intuition and cemented a much-flawed relationship where I stayed for years.

We married a little more than a year later despite a pushback from my family. We started dating in August, my father passed away on Christmas Eve that same year and we were married the following October.

Most of the hopes and dreams were mine. From buying a house to starting a family, they were all things I dreamed about and made happen. I had to take the lead and push for things as my spouse lived in a day-to-day mentality.

I was always looking ahead and striving for more. I quit the diner and returned to a professional job, making a good salary with a multitude of benefits. We bought a house in a great neighborhood and shortly thereafter I was diagnosed with Non-Hodgkins Lymphoma. This was the same disease that took my father's life a few years prior. This would put any hopes of having children off the table temporarily if not permanently or, so I was told.

Chapter 4 The Big C

Having Cancer is a real mind F***. From bone marrow testing, that is beyond painful, surgery, chemotherapies, hair loss and feeling sick. Mentally you are trying to wrap your mind around the fact that you could die, which can be overwhelming. I have always handled things bravely and kept my insecurities to myself. A strong front was my persona, and it really was done unintentionally. You do what you must.

People were amazed at my positive attitude. It was not something I chose; it was just who I was and still am to this day.

I was working a full-time job and only missed 1 day the entire year. I would work most of the day, drive into the city of Philadelphia by myself, get Chemotherapy and drive home. My spouse never went as he really could not take time off work. The nausea the following day is no joke. I was given high doses of prednisone to counteract the effects of the chemicals that would allow me to continue the next day. My hair loss was devastating to say the least. Most of my hair fell out within one day necessitating the wearing of a wig, which I hated. On my first day sporting my fresh look, my employer was taking head shots for a company directory. I was mortified.

That year was difficult, but the positive aspect was the purchase of our first home. My hair eventually grew back, about a year later. Scans that were routinely taken showed that all results were clear, and I was cancer free. I had dodged the bullet and never wanted to have to go through that again. I never thought I would have to endure that torture again; boy was I wrong. Unfortunately, in 2012 another form of Cancer revealed itself. My oldest child, a daughter graduated high school that year and the twins are now 14 years old.

Chapter 5 Not Again

After many years of stressful ones at that, I went for my routine mammogram. I was told immediately that an ultrasound was needed for additional radiology as something was amiss. This resulted in needing a needle biopsy on my left breast. I will await the results for several days.

While working a later shift I received a phone call from the radiologist advising me that I had breast cancer. I was dumbfounded as I never expected that result. I emailed my boss immediately and advised that I had to leave work as I could not function. I cried the whole way home as it was unbelievable that I would have to do this again. After an appointment with my oncologist, I learned that I would need a lumpectomy, chemotherapy, and radiation.

I had the surgery within a brief time. The tumor was dead center, deep behind the nipple. To rule out lymph node involvement I had a procedure just prior to the surgery where they inject dye that can be traced throughout the lymphatic system. The node in my arm pit would also be removed as a precaution. I had tremendous pain upon awakening after the surgery and severe nausea from the anesthesia. The node biopsy came back negative. The deformity from this surgery haunted me for many years as I was severely dented and uneven.

Chemotherapy was difficult but necessary. I had treatments every 3 weeks for several months followed by a month or two break before radiation treatments every day for a month. I took time off work on Fridays for my chemo treatments but changed my work hours to accommodate the radiation schedule and did not miss any time. Many years later I remain cancer free, however I am sometimes haunted by the thoughts of it returning. A cancer patient knows that at any time things can change quite suddenly and you always remain on guard.

The following year my daughter decided to move to Florida to pursue an online relationship she had developed with another woman. The actual move nearly ripped my heart out as we would be separated by 1200 miles (about 1931.21 km). One of the most difficult things I ever did in my life, with uncontrollable tears, was to board a plane to travel to Florida to ensure she got settled as she drove to Florida in her car packed for her new life.

Five weeks later the relationship would end, and she would return home.

Chapter 6 My Survival

My life was stressful. Working Full time, taking care of 3 kids and a single home is no easy feat. Add to that the boy's father was commuting 150 miles per day to work, which left him absent and exhausted. From frequent school meetings for IEPS, after school activities, sports, homework, getting everyone fed and to school on time the juggling of the kids and the house was taking a toll. I was overwhelmed. I never complained, just did what had to be done.

My coping mechanism was not healthy. Saturday became my excessive drinking day, often beginning at lunch time and going till late at night. I could relax, sort of, or at least numb the anxiety. I drank a lot, initially beer and later switched to Vodka. I had access to stimulants and indulged regularly to keep ahead of the effects of the alcohol and party for many hours. Eventually this grew old, and I gave it up in search of a healthier lifestyle, but it got me through. The same cannot be said of the kids' father as he indulged from the day we met and still does to this day.

I began to feel my marriage's decline, which resulted in many drunken arguments. I felt like I was changing, and my partner was not. I no longer felt in love but stuck in the marriage, as 2 incomes were needed to maintain our lifestyle and I did not want the kids to live through a divorce. We frequently argued over the discipline of the kids, Dad wanted to haul off and hit them. I was not raised that way, so I disagreed. Dad felt he was entitled to respect and yet he did not understand that respect is earned. His outbursts surely would not bring him the respect he thought he deserved. In fact, his behavior had the opposite effect. Years later he had not changed and had not been able or willing to understand the connection between actions and consequences. His children do not look up to him today and if anything, they look down on him.

This became a big divide in the marriage. In retrospect I was wrong as I delayed making necessary changes. My spouse became increasingly frustrated and angry frequently referring to me as a "cunt" during arguments and then replaying his displeasure to the children referring to me in the same way. It was unsettling to hear the children relay their conversations to me and made me sad to know they had to hear the level of negativity and anger that spewed from their father's mouth. He really has no control over his anger hence his coping mechanisms remain ineffective.

Drugs and alcohol are escapes from life. They do nothing to help you deal with your stress. In fact, they add to it the guilt of indulging as well as the effects on your body are depressive. It becomes a vicious cycle and one that takes strength and determination to resist. It also does not help when your partner continues to partake, and you have access at any time. Once I quit partying I never went back. I also gave up smoking around the same time. Why not eliminate everything at once? I was starting to feel like it was time for me, and I wanted to live a healthier life. I needed to focus on myself and become a better role model. My health suffered because of my choices, and I wanted to live a long healthy life for my children and myself.

Chapter 7 Fast Forward

The twins are now 18. They are graduating from Cyber school, thank goodness for that. The question is now what? My daughter, 4 years older, had enrolled in college and was trying to find her way in life. Neither of the twins had any desire to continue an education of any sort. They are staying up late at night gaming. There is some lawn work being done for income and small jobs for neighbors. Ryan is ready to pursue a military career as his lifelong dream.

James has become more anxiety ridden and less likely to want to leave the house let alone his bedroom. He begins eating all his meals in his bedroom where dirty dishes pile up for days with remnants of leftover food. He does not shower very often, and his effect is concerning. He has anxiety medication but has stopped taking it.

We have always taken family vacations in the summer, and we are set to go to a Pocono retreat in a modern cabin that sits on a lake. As the men love to fish and there are nearby shopping outlets there is something for everyone to do. Deposits have been made and its nearing time to go. James does not want to go. I had never left him alone before and I am sad that he could potentially miss a fun time. His decision was made so we reluctantly went. A close family neighbor agrees to check in on him which helps to relieve my worries.

Once there we fish, shop, go out on the lake and paddle around. My daughter and I book a horseback ride and the men book an off-road ATV excursion. On the day before these events, we head out to a local go kart arena for some fun. I stay back and watch from the stands. As I am looking at Ryan coming around the bend his facial expression is concerning. At the same time, he begins to seize and drives head on into a retaining wall. All I can think of is not again.

Ryan's life dream has been to go into the military, and he had even spoken with a recruiter. All he had talked about since he was little was his desire to join the military. I now know that his dreams will not become a reality as having epilepsy is not permitted in the armed services. My heart breaks for him. An ambulance comes and he refuses transport. Ryan complains all the way back to the cabin of severe low back pain and a headache. He is up most of the night in severe pain and I locate a walk-in clinic that has X-ray on site to visit the next day. They do not X-ray him indicating that it is not necessary and provide at home exercises as well as medications which we fill in immediately.

The ATV excursion had to be canceled. I spent an entire day setting up appointments for specialists and making calls to the insurance carrier to confirm out of town treatment. The ride home is painful for Ryan. His pain does dissipate some over time and life goes on. We are anxious to see the specialists and get some answers.

A couple of months later while seeing the family doctor for another issue, Ryan mentions his back pain so his doctor orders a back X-ray. X-rays revealed a fracture in his lumbar spine sustained during the go cart crash. He is immediately given a referral to an Orthopedic doctor who prescribes exercises and a back brace to be worn continuously for several months.

The neurologist is great and very personable, which is good. Ryan likes him. He prescribes a generic seizure medication and orders tests. With the 6-

year gap in seizures, it is said that more than likely Ryan has juvenile myoclonic epilepsy. The specialist also advises that there are more effective medications which have more side effects and may not interact well with the other medications that Ryan takes so we will try this generic one to start.

One night some weeks later, I was in my room about to go to sleep, and I heard a loud crash coming from Ryan's room. With an older home and wooden floors anything that hits the floors is heard throughout the house. This was loud and worrisome. I ran to his bedroom door to find it locked. His brother appeared from his room next door, and we quickly realized that something was going on in the room and Ryan was not answering. James kicked the door in, and we found Ryan on the floor seizing himself, having fallen from his computer chair.

This was one of many ongoing seizures that Ryan endured throughout the next year or so. Having seen a neurologist at one point it was clear that something needed to change. His seizures became more frequent over several months. Often, he would fall during the seizures and injure himself.

After several seizures, sometimes more than once in a week, it was evident that he needed a change in medication. It became a constant worry as you were always waiting for another seizure and never knowing when it would happen. You were always on edge and praying he would not get hurt while falling. His medication was eventually changed and thankfully he has now been seizure free for several years. He has been able to get a driver's license, after losing his permit due to a seizure, and remains healthy and independent. He will have to remain on medication for the rest of his life.

Chapter 8 FBI

There is nothing like hearing pounding on your front door early in the morning only to look out the window seeing a light beam coming from a gun aimed at your head. The front yard is smattered with FBI agents and wet leaves, and they are all yelling at me to open the door. The dog is barking loudly and all I can think is that they may shoot her. The kids had been sleeping and I was getting ready for work. Once I open the door, there are many more agents as the house is surrounded. All exits are covered as they advance inside.

Once they are inside, they methodically go from room to room clearing each area. The kids have already woken up with all the commotion. We are all separated, and the dog is banished to the basement. Initially I was concerned for Ryan as he was up too late and needed his sleep. I am fearing another seizure will rear its ugly head as lack of sleep and the stress of the experience may contribute to this occurring.

The kid's dad has already left for work, so I am dealing with this alone. I called out of work and answered questions as best as I could. This event lasted several hours as each one of us was questioned and all electronics in the house were confiscated. The target of this investigation is baby A.

We have just recently been advised, I believe 6 or so years later, that James has been cleared of any wrongdoing and all equipment will be returned if wanted but must be wiped. So, we are about to receive 18 out of date phones, laptops, and gaming consoles. Most of the items have been disassembled and are returned in a dysfunctional condition. Funny how that works, we are significantly affected and yet he was innocent.

The cost of these items was borne by the parents, and we are the most affected as items returned are trash. I am talking about expensive phones, laptops, and gaming consoles. Certainly, initially worth thousands of dollars. Not to mention they are all outdated.

Chapter 9 Reality

The boys are growing up. There is no interest in furthering their education. There must be a plan as I cannot support them forever. They both apply for dishwashing jobs at a senior living facility and are hired. At least it is something but as suspected it does not last long. One got fired and the other walked out, which does not surprise me.

Up to this point the boys have not ventured out much and have little to no social life as they attended cyber school and lost contact with their school peers. A little money in their pockets and a sense of needing more they reconnect with a group of guys from their high school class.

Multiple nights of drinking and partying ensued as one of their friends clearly lived in the party mansion. A constant flow of young adults visited the house day and night. At first only James went but he urged Ryan to join yet he was hesitant. It was not until James got a steady girlfriend and stopped going that Ryan started going.

Sometime later James took a job delivering pizzas and bought a car. It seemed that neither of their lives were going anywhere as there was no end goal or plan for their futures. James is extremely talented with web design, but any type of formal education turns him off. Ryan has built a few computers by this time and has an affinity for it. He has also been able to reapply for his license having waited the required 6 months following his seizures.

James has always had big dreams. He also wants the best of everything and has an eye for expensive things. Unfortunately, he does not have the means to live such a lifestyle and is not realistic with his dreams. One day he is going to apply for a solid job with benefits and the next day he is going to go back to food service. He needs to plan and stick to it. I am not sure what must happen for him to get on track.

Ryan is seeing the writing on the wall and realizes that he might need an education to advance in his life. He wants to pursue additional education with cybersecurity and eventually he enrolls in the local community college where he did very well, graduates with honors and moves onto another school for his bachelor's degree. He is pursuing that degree now.

Chapter 10 The Fall

In January 2022 I awoke to yelling. It was around midnight and as I focused, I realized it was the boys, Dad. As he had slept on the Living room sofa for years, he was near to the emergency. He was in the front foyer hovering over someone yelling that we needed an ambulance as another seizure had occurred. I immediately assumed it was Ryan but soon learned that it was James. Since Ryan had been diagnosed with Epilepsy, I was sure it was him. James had never had a seizure.

As I descended the steps, I saw James's slides sitting halfway down the steps. It became clear he had begun to seize while on the steps and fell down the steps from about the halfway point. His shoes remained at the point from which he lost consciousness and began to seize. Seizures are horrific to witness. The jerking movements are followed by an unsettling period of deep groans unlike anything you can duplicate or have heard before. The sound is guttural as it is the time where your brain is trying to reset.

Once coherent James is in pain. Ambulance and police arrived, and we learn that he has potential fractures from the fall and will need hospital transport. As we are still under Covid restrictions the hospital will not allow me to stay with him. I am forced to go home and wait for phone calls to update me. James calls frequently so I end up being up most of the night. He is finally discharged around 5:00am so I go pick him up. He is diagnosed with a slight concussion, a fractured left wrist, and a sprained right shoulder.

Initially the wrist fracture is thought to be minor, and the shoulder heals. I scheduled a neurology appointment. James will now need seizure medication as well. He will not be able to drive for 6 months and cannot work as he drives for his employment. He has a car payment and credit card bills. He is due in court that morning for traffic violations. Obviously, he will not be able to go so I called and plead with the court for a continuance which they grant.

The next month I am awakened again to pounding on the front door around 5:00 am. It is the police who have come to arrest James. He is being charged with distribution of a controlled substance and is facing 5 federal charges. Off he goes. He will see the judge that day when a $75,00 bail is set. If we pay 10%, he will be released before his court date. I leave and go to work as I had before. It has been one thing after another with James.

His car had been reposed several days before and I had maxed out my credit cards to pay the back payments and get the car released. He had stayed all night and into a second night when he had the seizure. He was up gaming with friends. He was not taking care of himself or his responsibilities and was making bad choices. Anything to make a dollar.

James's dad contacted his father as we did not have the kind of money that was needed for his bail. The arrangements were made, and he was released later that day. In the meantime, his wrist complaints continued as did his headache along with the charges and involvement in the legal system. His attorney helped him avoid jail time and placed him in an outpatient drug program that required attendance 3 days per week, a sponsor, and evening community Alon on meetings every night. He would also have weekly meetings with his probation officer and be drug tested. Frequent court appearances and one-on-one counseling were also required.

In April James saw an Orthopedic surgeon who specialized in hand and wrist injuries. The cat scan results were concerning. He would require extensive surgery to include rods and pins and a second surgery several months later to remove the hardware. As James fears being put to sleep, he opts to remain awake for the surgery, having a nerve block, so he does not feel anything. He will not be able to take any narcotics for pain due to his drug treatment program and seems fine with that until the pain hits that night. It would become a long road to recovery with the second surgery and therapy and one year later he was still not up to speed.

Since he had not worked in over a year and debt was mounting, he decided to file for bankruptcy to get a fresh start. Meanwhile he has filed for disability to be initially denied and is now awaiting appeal. He will clearly lose his car, as it has been in a shop for over a year with a blown engine, and paying for repairs is impossible.

Chapter 11 The Separation

My lack of happiness went back many years. I knew I was in a loveless marriage and hated where I was at. I began dieting and exercising routinely and over a year and a half lost slightly over 40 pounds. My confidence was growing. I had been out of work from my professional job due to downsizing and after a severance was offered by my employer. Now I am finally able to focus more on myself. I took a mindless job at a local grocery store after not working for a year or so only to tear my rotator cuff and eventually need surgery.

Following my recovery I returned to the same employer, a different job, continuing to care for myself and searching for who I was and what would make me happy. It is only appropriate that as I sit her authoring this book on the balcony of my own apartment I am now finally alone. Yes, I had to get out and find tranquility. The explosiveness and roller coaster ride with the spouse had become too much. I am now in the process of finding my happiness and determining what I want in my life. I am no longer living in an unstable, toxic environment.

This was the scariest and most awkward thing I had to do, more so than going through chemotherapy. The spouse had never written a check, paid a bill, managed a bank account, or handled any online transactions. I initially told him I wanted a separation in the fall of 2021. He stated he would have to get his shit together as he knew the gravity of the situation. In all honesty I was already done. He never did make any attempts to clean up his act so there was less guilt.

I stayed at the house in a separate state until I signed a lease and moved out in August 2022. I told all my family members about my decision to leave. The planning and calculating took tedious calculation as I wanted to split the financial responsibilities evenly. When I finally sat and calculated the earnings, I was shocked to see we were about even. As he kept more than half his earnings to himself things were about to change drastically. I split the bills evenly making sure there was plenty left over for out-of-pocket expenses like gas, lunches, entertainment or whatever. I pushed for him to open a bank account and moved his paycheck to direct deposit in his account.

The spouse never notified his family until the day of my move. He was in denial, hoping I would not leave. Thanks to the help of my daughter things have fallen into place. All three children remain at the house with the ex and have adjusted to my absence. I do miss the kids and try to spend time with them weekly. I also miss living in a single home as apartment living just does not compare but it was a tradeoff I had to make and would not change.

Chapter 12 Rebirth

Not only was I extremely excited to depart my home of 32 years but I was anxious about the prospect of living alone. It was bittersweet as at times I missed the kids, and the loneliness was unavoidable. In retrospect it allowed me to do some deep soul searching as well as recover from years of emotional abuse. Leaving the kids in the environment caused a lot of guilt, but they were all adults and I had to do this for myself.

My work family's support helped me gather the strength to move forward. There were 3 special people in my life at that time who

supported me and enabled me to maintain the courage to move forward. One in particular frequently told me he was "proud" of me. To this day I am grateful for that friendship and the impact it had on my life. It is funny how certain people come into your life for a reason and unfortunate how they then leave.

One of the first things I did was to get a tattoo of a phoenix on my right shoulder. It truly represented my rebirth into a new life where I never heard the word "no" and could do whatever I wanted. I realized for several months that what I was searching for was peace. After living in a volatile environment, I had become someone I did not know. I was always on edge and ready to battle.

I moved to a town I lived in near my home before being married, walkable to the town center. The county seat had good shopping, great restaurants, and lots of events throughout the year.

I attended several events initially, by myself, which added to my loneliness. The apartment was nice and offered outdoor space with a balcony.

It took time to decompress and figure out what I wanted to do with my life. My job was becoming too physically demanding, hours were being cut and new management had made it an unpleasant environment. I also no longer had all the support that had been there so nothing there made me want to stay. I started looking for another job and quickly found one that checked all the boxes and accepted a new position.

Again, I am working at a physical job and have daily physical pain as I am getting older but still need an income to support myself. With a pension from my professional job and social security additional income is still needed. I am contributing to the household with groceries, paying for the cell phone and insurance bill. I also carry medical insurance for the family.

My social security came into play as I tore a rotator cuff which required surgery and extensive rehabilitation. The sad part is that I know what a torn rotator cuff feels like, and I am told that people who have one shoulder tear often have the other shoulder tear. I hope not! It required me to be out of work for an extended time, so I will have to keep my fingers crossed. My job requires lifting and reaching, both of which can cause this injury.

The summer has always been great for me, and it is even better now as I can do whatever I want without hearing a "no" with a thousand reasons as to why this trip or event is a bad idea. With money also being separate I have all the freedom I need. From trips to the shore, day events and summer excursions I am content. The kids are always up for adventures as well, so it works out.

The only negative is that the ex will tell the kids he feels "left out." He is meant to be left out as it is time for him to make his own memories with the kids and work on his relationships with them as they are not good. He has become increasingly needy and frequently battles with the kids over their lack of interaction with him. They do not want to interact and avoid him as much as possible. The kids know he is an addict and do not respect him. He also drinks too much so the weekends are difficult for them as he is usually half lit at midday and at home.

Throughout this time, I have taken more interest in my spirituality and learned about our divine counterparts and how they play a role in our daily lives. From archangels to synchronicities, it is a fascinating realm for which I have dug into evolving my consciousness. I am what they call a light worker as I have a positive outlook on life and spread myself among people who frequently need a hand to enlighten them and uplift themselves. I never realized how my positivity was so rare and that through that I have helped a lot of people. I can support people with unconditional love, never judging anyone. This thought process raises the environment for the entire collective.

Chapter 13 Spiritual Awakening

I believe that I had met my Twin Flame in my past. I met a man who has captured my attention like no other. I remember saying to him at one point you are the male version of me. I also remember early on him noticing my Chakra bracelets and going as far as removing one from my wrist and claiming it has its own. I had no idea at that time if Twin Flames shared a Chakra system or what they were.

Our contacts stopped suddenly, and it took a real toll on me. I felt like a part of me had been severed. Months later I am now learning about this dynamic and why it has had such a profound impact on me. He is on my mind constantly, but he must deal with his Karma and embark on his own spiritual journey before he can come forward. Twin Flames mirror each other's feelings.

Some Twin Flames remain separated for years on end. It is easy to become skeptical with so much time passing and not truly knowing how your twin really feels. There are times where I have felt that we communicate telepathically or have visits in my dreams but again time plays with your mind. Collective readings are for the masses and although insightful the information may not apply. Faith is essential as the feminine are supposed to attract not chase. You must release all to the Divine and await that timing.

You also must learn forgiveness for past hurts and learn to heal your own hurts. No one can do that for you and conceptualizing this can have an enormous impact on your journey. You may act by performing manifestations. That is a skill that takes practice and patience. You must feel as if your wish is already in your space and project the feelings that the wish would give you providing it is in your space. People often manifest abundance, love &

careers, in hopes of one day attaining that wish.

This entire process has awakened my spirituality and given me solace in reminding me that there are powers bigger than us. I have uncovered an ability to recognize signs and synchronicities sent by our spirits whether celestial or people who have passed on. As a light worker I have learned that my "job" in life is to help others and I can do this by connecting with spirit to help raise others up. Twin Flames share this responsibility once reunited. Twin Flames cannot be reunited until inner blocks are released and negative energy is removed. The Divine Feminine takes the lead as their spiritual side is more awakened.

If you ask for confirmation or signs from Spirit, you will get them. Unfortunately, we often miss these signs in the hustle and bustle of life. I am Learning to slow down and try to be more aware of my surroundings including taking a lot of time for myself. Part of this process involves pouring into yourself to become more whole. Signs and synchronicities are the spirit's way of showing you that you are on the right path.

Grounding with nature is important as it helps to bring you back into focus with life and what is important. You must also surrender to the Divine for your life path. Spirit will protect you and guide you into that direction based on Divine timing. Patience is key as well as having faith and believing that your guides will always have your best interest at heart. There is a lot going on in the celestial realm that we cannot see so we must trust.

With time and focus on myself I am certain my union will occur. The Divine will not allow my Twin to come forward if he is where he was when we last encountered each other as he was not healed. He also served to unearth my insecurities and put me on a path of healing and entering my own awakening. I knew when I met him that he had great qualities and would one day bring us both peace and happiness, something we have failed to attain at this point in our lives. It is going to be monumental!

Chapter 14 The Final Chapter

As I sit on my balcony, I realize that I am finally at peace with my life and who

I have become. It took a while to realize what affect my past living situation had on me. I lived in a very unhealthy environment for many years. Initially I would try to keep the peace but eventually I became increasingly angry as I realized that some people cannot evolve and look at things realistically. People have limits and mindsets that refuse to grow. Love turns to hate and resentment where there is no turning back and a lack of trust. This traumatic lifestyle truly took a toll on me, where a lot of emotions were buried.

I have changed a lot over this last year, spending a lot of time in solitude and soul searching. I have learned to focus on myself and be my biggest cheerleader. I am grateful for so many things now.

I have also learned to speak my appreciation out into the universe. From my new home, my kids, my piece of mind, my new job, the beautiful air we breathe as well as the wonderful opportunities to travel and finally be the person I was truly meant to be, I am forever grateful. The delay in my journey was no one's fault but my own based on the choices I have made and the people I have surrounded myself with.

I have learned so much about human nature and how we relate to the outer world and the effects it can have on our lives. It is amazing to comprehend that what we say can become reality and to know that one individual can raise the vibration of the entire world. As we have positive interactions with people, they in turn do the same with others. It creates a massive positive domino effect.

I am not sure what the next chapter of my life will be, but I am hopeful that it will be peaceful and inspiring. I love new adventures and hope to share my life with someone who also wants the same type of coexistence as I do. Having lived with so much negativity for so many years resulted in a lower vibrational world of being stuck with limiting choices and a lack of growth. I have always said that "everything happens for a reason" and my life embodies this sentiment. In addition, we all need to embrace the thought that "where there is a will there is a way."

Having survived cancer twice, leaving a dysfunctional marriage, dealing with drug abuse, raising children, twins as well as a singleton, two with medical and emotional disabilities, it has been challenging to say the least. You cannot give up or give in as the life you want can be obtained and you can truly live in peace one day. The house that never sleeps was a never-ending exhausting journey but one I would not change for the world. Without that house I would not be where I am today. Keep faith and believe!